I0425442

The Ultimate keto Diet Recipes For Beginners

Delicious Ketogenic Diet Meals To Lose Weight, Fat Burning, Low Carb, Nutrition And Reverse Disease

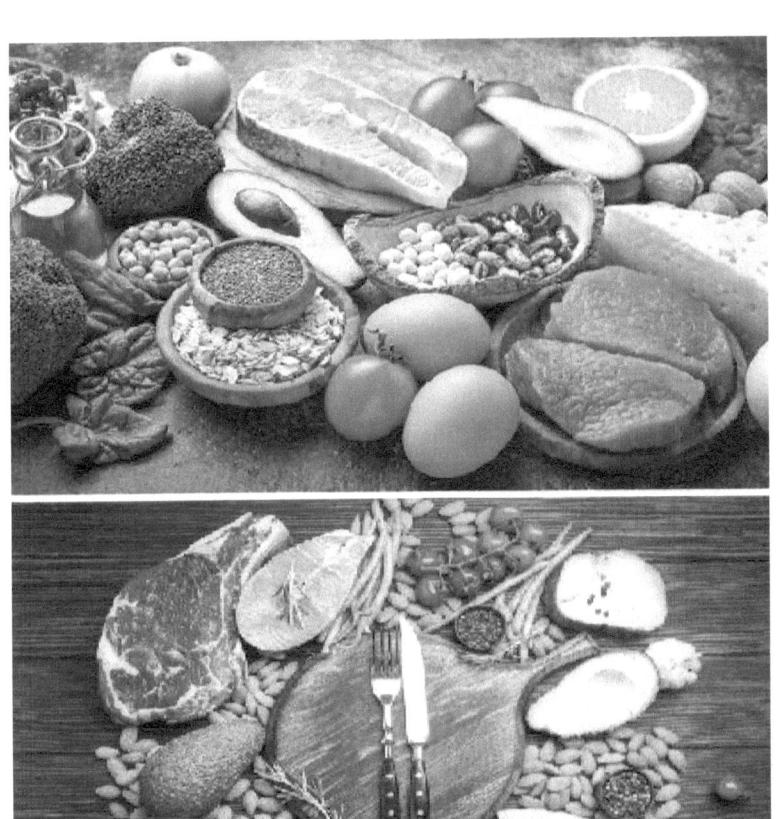

Table of Contents

Introduction

The ketogenic diet is an aggravated form of low-carbohydrate diet that has many friends, especially among athletes. Carbohydrate-containing foods such as bread and pasta are all deleted on the ketogenic diet. Instead, high-fat foods are on the menu. So the body should take advantage of the so-called ketosis . But what does it actually mean when you become ketogenic nourished? The term derived from ketosis, a metabolic process in which the body gets its energy from fat instead of sugar and carbohydrates. These are usually the first sources of energy for the body. However, if it gets neither sugar nor carbohydrates, which it can convert to glucose, it resorts instead to the fat deposits in the body. The brain uses these formed so-called ketones or ketone bodies for energy supply.

Brief History of ketogenic Diet

The ketogenic diet is a direct successor to the fast, also called ketosis. Being fasted since the beginning of humanity. First of all, due to the food shortage in the cold winter months at the time of our earliest ancestors. Later, for example, the Greeks have rediscovered the many health benefits of fasting and actively fasted to fight disease. To date, moderate fasting is considered to be healthy for the human body. The Ketogene diet is a form of fasting, as long-lasting sugary and starchy foods are avoided. This diet is strongly based on the original diet of the earliest humans.

In 1996, the American film "First do not harm" was broadcast. The film tells the story of a boy suffering from epilepsy, who is given a strict ketogenic diet to fight his illness in a special clinic. The film was broadcast in Germany under the name "While there is still hope". At the same time, for example, the great weight-reducing effect of the ketogenic diet became known, as a result of which this diet suddenly enjoyed great popularity.

Even today, the ketogenic diet is enjoying great popularity due to its weight-reducing and health-promoting effect. Not least because today the relationships between a low-calorie diet and the cure of diseases due to countless studies can be better understood. The ketogenic diet is so popular today, because it can be overweight in a healthy way and without being reduced to starvation.

Different types of ketogenic diet

The SKD, Standard Ketogenic Diet , was designed in the 1920s for the treatment of severe epilepsy. This diet is isocaloric, protein normal, high in fat and low in carbohydrates. The goal is the state of ketosis, in which the energy is produced by ketone bodies. By a greatly increased fat burning the three ketone bodies acetoac-etate, beta-hydroxybutyrate and acetone are formed. The positive effects of short-term ketosis were initially used for medical purposes and had not been designed for the purpose of weight loss. Carbohydrate consumption is reduced to a minimum to help the body cleanse and detoxify.

The CKD, Cyclical Ketogenic Diet , is particularly suitable for professional body-builders, since the basic requirement for the success of this diet is a high training volume. This is especially suitable for athletes who can not increase their muscle volume through the TKD. Athletes can get a huge boost in performance through the CKD. Here are two cycles suitable for training. Cycle 1 is the total renunciation of carbohydrates for 5-6 days. At this time the body is in ketosis. In the second cy-cle, the refleed takes place for 1-2 days, whereby the mucous glycogen stores are filled up by a massive supply of carbohydrates. Through regular and high-intensity training, these reserves are used up again before the next refeed.

The TKD, Targeted Ketogenic Diet , is especially designed for athletes who want to push their limits. By eating carbohydrates just before the workout, you can achieve a short-term boost in performance without interrupting ketosis for a longer period of time. Before the workout, 25-50g of high glycemic carbohydrates are consumed. The muscles thus have glycogen available and can be further developed without the fat is applied. This form should be introduced only after at least 12 weeks of successful standard ketogenic diet.

The high-protein Ketogenic Diet is particularly suitable for athletes who are in a phase of muscle building. In addition to the 20-50g carbohydrates daily, a large amount of protein in the form of fish, meat, soy or synthetic building materials is added to the ketogenic diet. This provides the optimal basis for muscle building and a long-lasting satiety.

The LCT diet, long-chain triglycerides , is a special form of ketogenic diet that provides a dietary composition of fats and carbohydrates / proteins in the ratio 4: 1 or 3: 1. The LCT-containing fats and oils from the diet have a high energy density and provide the body around 10 percent more energy than other fats. They are degraded more slowly and thus ensure a long-term satiety. This form of ketogenic diet is good for losing weight. The long-chain fatty acids have an energy content of 9.2 kcal.

The MCT diet, medium-chain triglycerices , provides above all for a focused intake of medium-chain fatty acids. These have a lower energy density of 8.3 kcal instead of 9.2 kcal compared to long-chain fatty acids. They are therefore very ketogenic and are broken down faster in the body. It is consumed at a lower total fat content more fat. About 60 percent of energy is derived from medium-chain fatty acids, 10 percent from proteins and 20 percent from carbohydrates. The advantage of this diet is that a more varied diet can be created due to the increased levels of protein and carbohydrates. This diet is equally suitable for losing weight as the LCT diet.

The Atkins Dietwas published in the 1970s by Robert Atkins and commercialized from 1989 by the company Atkins Nutritionals Inc. commercially. In the first phase of the diet, which extends over the first two weeks, not more than 5g of carbohydrates should be consumed daily. Phases 2 and 3 involve more carbohydrates with steady weight loss. The fourth phase is then the final nutritional plan, which should ensure a stable ideal weight. Basically, the consumption of proteins and fats is highly considered. Due to the lack of carbohydrates, the body is to reduce the energy of the body's own fat. In addition, over the entire period dietary supplements, synthetic vitamins and synthetic minerals are to be taken for optimal nutrition.

The principles of ketogenic diet

The Ketogene diet aims to provide an optimal nutrient intake for the body with low exposure to disease-promoting substances. Here, the needs of the human body are oriented, which have hardly changed since early humanity. An adaptation of the diet is necessary because of changes in access and variety of food. For today's humans, there are no more natural fasting periods and a maximum oversupply of fast food, high-carbohydrate diet and high-sugar ready meals. This diet favors the emergence of diseases such as cancer or multiple sclerosis, to name but two.

The basic ingredients of the ketogenic diet are nutritious vegetables, high quality vegetable fats, nuts, seeds, meat, fish and animal products. The basis for this is the fresh and independent preparation of meals, in order to supply the body with as many vital nutrients and minerals as possible on a daily basis, which are necessary for the defense and control of diseases. A positive side effect is the simultaneous weight reduction. The ketogens diet does not provide any sugary, pre-made or industrially heavily processed foods.

This favors the condition of ketosis. Here, the metabolic state of the body is completely changed because no more energy can be gained from carbohydrates. Thus, the body is forced to use the energy stored in fat cells and to gain energy from other fuels. For example, from the ketones produced in the liver. This condition occurs when less than 50g of carbohydrate is supplied over an extended period of time. The ketosis takes place mainly in the liver. This process produces ketone bodies that provide the body with energy. In ketosis, the substances acetone, acetoacetic acid and beta-hydroxybutanoic acid are produced, which can lead to a fruity body odor. If the ketosis persists for a longer period, excess fat is broken down, which leads to weight loss. At the same time, the cancerous cells or other harmful cells are deprived of their livelihood due to the lack of sugar.Over a longer period of time, the body gets used to using fat as an energy resource.

How and why does the ketogenic diet work?

To get started with the ketogenic diet, it is necessary to think in advance, as it is not advisable to stop carbohydrates. Creating a nutritional plan for the first few weeks makes sense to avoid food insecurity and minimize stress.

In the first 14 days there is a change of the body and a restriction of the carbohydrates adapted to the own well-being. The body and the psyche get used to the change in diet and the new diet becomes part of everyday life. After this time, most of the state of ketosis is reached. The condition is not measurable in terms of well-being or symptoms. By measuring the ketosis, certainty about the state of ketosis can be obtained. Also, by measuring the ketone body in the blood, the diet can be further optimized and adapted and averted a possible ketoacidosis. Ketosticks that detect ketosis in the urine are helpful for this. These test strips are actually designed for diabetics, but can be purchased over the counter in pharmacies.

However, these test strips do not provide accurate information on the state of ketosis and are therefore only suitable for the initial detection of the use of ketosis. For athletes who are passionate about ketogenic nutrition or sick people, the electronic device Ketonix, which measures acetone in the breath, can be used. Thus, the progress of the ketosis can be measured. By regular blood measurements, the concentration of beta-hydroxybutyrates in the blood can be detected and thus also specify a very detailed status of ketosis. However, such an accurate measurement is not necessary when performing the ketogenic diet for the purpose of muscle building or weight loss, but is specifically directed to the needs of sick people.

- The ketosis

Ketosis is the desired state of the ketogenic diet. Ketosis burns a lot of fat without feeling hungry. As soon as carbohydrates are no longer available to the body over a longer period of time, the body's own fat is burned and used to generate energy. At the same time ketone bodies are created in the liver for energy production. These ketone bodies are the source of energy during ketosis instead of glucose. These ketone bodies are made from the molecules acetoacetate, 3-hydroxybutyrate and acetone. As the carbohydrates are split from the pancreas using the hormone insulin, the production of insulin during ketosis becomes unnecessary or extremely limited. This results in a stable blood pressure. Humans are by nature "fat burners", why the condition of ketosis, in which fat is burned, healthy. In particular, a light ketosis, without the total renunciation of carbohydrates, is beneficial for the control and prevention of diseases.

In order to stay in the ketosis, it is important to avoid carbohydrates, so that the energy can continue to take place through the ketone body and excess fat can be broken down and can not be rebuilt. The intake of carbohydrates would cause the energy production from ketone bodies to be interrupted and energy to be recovered from the carbohydrates.

This does not mean that carbohydrates should never be consumed again. In the beginning, it is important to abstain completely from carbohydrates for 3-5 days in order to start the ketosis. However, depending on your age and physical condition, it can take up to 6 months for ketosis to set in. This should be checked with appropriate aids such as Ketosticks. Then you can consume up to 0.8 g of carbohydrates per kilogram of body weight without ending the ketosis.

During ketosis, the foods mentioned below should be consumed. It is important to take 3-4 hours between meals to eat high-fat foods. In addition, the diet should provide daily 30-50 g of protein per day.

Tips to stay in stressful everyday life in the ketosis are well-prepared shopping lists, the mucking out of food that is not beneficial for the ketosis and prepared snacks such as meatballs, hard-boiled eggs, almonds.

If necessary, bratwurst, Kassler and Bifi are good to quench hunger in a ketogenic way. A glass of water with lemon juice and stevia helps against the cravings in between. In order to be well prepared at home even in stressful times, it is advisable to stock frozen products such as shrimps or vegetables.

It is fundamentally important that ketosis can only be realized for healthy people and under medical supervision.

3 Tips for Success on the Ketogenic Diet

ketogenic diets are still very highly regarded in many circles as effective, maintainable weight loss diets. Below are a few tips to maximize your success on a ketogenic diet.

1.) Drink tons of water.

While on a ketogenic diet, your body has a hard time retaining as much water as it needs, so staying properly hydrated is absolutely essential. Many experts recommend that men intake a minimum of 3 liters of beverages each day, while the figure for women is 2.2 liters daily. A good indicator of proper hydration is the color of your urine. If your urine is clear or light yellow, you're most likely properly hydrated. Keep a bottle of water with you everywhere you go!

2.) Don't forget the fat!

Simply put, our bodies need fuel to function. When we limit our carbohydrate intake, especially to levels that induce ketosis, our bodies need an alternate fuel source. Since protein is not an efficient source of energy, our bodies turn to fat. Any fat you eat while in ketosis is used for energy, making it very difficult to store fat while in ketosis. Choose healthy, unsaturated fats as often as possible: foods like avocados, olives, nuts, and seeds are ideal.

3) Be patient.

While the ketogenic diet is known for rapid weight loss, especially in the early stages of the diet, weight loss is always a slow, time-consuming process. Don't freak out if the scale doesn't show weight loss, or shows slight weight increases, for a few days. Your weight varies day-to-day (and throughout the day) based upon a number of factors. Don't forget to use metrics like how your clothes fit or body measurements to see progress beyond what the scale shows.

Foods to consume in the ketogenic diet

- meat

Meat, as it contains little or no carbohydrates and a lot of proteins and fats. Red meats such as steaks and ham are great, as are chicken and turkey.

- dairy products

Dairy products may be included in large quantities in the nutrition plan. Above all, butter, cream and cheese are harmless usable foods. Yogurt should be as fat and unsweetened as possible, so that it complies with the principles of ketogenic nutrition.

- eggs

Eggs contain no carbohydrates and are very rich in protein. They are incredibly versatile, making them a perfect base food for the ketogenic diet.

- vegetable

Vegetables are a cornerstone of the ketogenic diet. Especially green vegetables, tomatoes and onions have a high nutrient content and a low carbohydrate content and are therefore indispensable. Avocados have a high fat content and are therefore a great and widely used element in the kitchen of the ketogenic diet.

- fish

Fish, especially greasy species such as mackerel, tuna, salmon or trout. These species often contain a high proportion of the incredibly healthy omega-3 fatty acid, which is very important for the ketogenic diet.

- Nuts and seeds

Nuts and seeds contain natural proteins and fats, making them the ideal companion to the ketogenic diet. In addition to walnuts, chia seeds , almonds and pumpkin seeds are recommended without hesitation. Nuts and seeds are particularly suitable as a companion for baking, in smoothies or as a snack. On the positive side, they hardly contain carbohydrates.

- spices

Of course, spices should not be missing in the Ketogene kitchen. However, here are fresh spices to be preferred because, for example, the marinade of pre-marinated meat spices mixed with sugar.

- oils

Oils, as fats are a basis of ketogenic nutritional form. High quality oils such as virgin olive oil, coconut oil or avocado oil

Foods to avoid

- cereals

Grains can get up to 70 percent carbs. Therefore, it is important to avoid the intake of small portions of rice, pasta or bread so as not to interrupt the ketosis.

- fruit

Fruit contains a high amount of fructose. Although this natural fructose is healthy in moderation, it causes ketosis to be broken.

- legumes

Legumes like lentils, beans or peas are high in carbohydrates, so it's important to avoid them as well.

- potatoes

Potatoes and potato products such as dumplings, French fries, dumplings or the like contain a high percentage of carbohydrates.

- convenience foods

Ready meals usually contain in addition to flavor enhancers also a lot of sugar. These have no place in the ketogenic diet.

- Alcoholic drinks

Alcoholic beverages such as vodka or whiskey do not contain carbohydrates, but alcohol is a foreign substance for the body. When alcohol is consumed, it is first broken down and energy is lost. Since the general health benefit of alcohol is questionable, it is recommended during the phase of ketogenic diet to refrain from it.

Ketogenic Diet : Side effects and hazards

There are some risk groups for which the ketogenic diet is not suitable. It can also lead to unwanted side effects, if the diet is not introduced gently.

- The risk groups

While the ketogenic diet is used primarily for improving children's health in the US, dietary ketogens are not recommended for healthy children. For example, physicians warn of growth delays and devastating development delays due to deficiency symptoms. Pregnant and nursing women are also strongly advised against ketogenic diets.Physicians expressly warns against ketogenic nutrition during pregnancy. Even with gestational diabetes, dietary kinetics can cause extreme harm to unborn baby growth.

People with gallbladder disease should avoid the ketogenic diet due to the increased intake of fats. The bile produces gall fluid to get the fats from the food. A diseased bile may not be able to cope with the amount of fat ingested, which can cause nausea and complications. However, people without gallbladder self-experimentation with the ketogenic diet and reported positive results.

There may be a connection with a low carbohydrate diet and the formation of kidney stones. However, the connection has not been sufficiently researched for a substantiated statement. Most people can eat a ketogenic diet without getting kidney stones. However, people who are prone to kidney stones should refrain from the ketogenic diet.

If the function of the pancreas is disturbed, ie there is an exocrine pancreatic insufficiency, then not enough enzymes can be produced for the digestion. Symptoms of this can be unhealthy bowel movements, abdominal cramps, bloating, bloating and weight loss. Since exocrine pancreatic insufficiency primarily affects the breakdown of fats, the high fat-based ketogenic diet is not tolerated for people with exocrine pancreatic insufficiency. It can come to a deficiency from the fats won vitamins A, D, E or K. Depending on the severity of the disease, carbohydrate intake is essential.

People who suffer from anorexia or other eating disorders should not carry out the ketogenic diet. Especially with anorexia, ie reduced appetite, in combination with a ketogenic diet can lead to an undersupply of essential vitamins and energy. Even with other eating disorders such as bulimia is not advised to ketogenic diet, as it can also come here to a deficiency of vitamins and energy-supplying substances. The ketogenic diet is especially about the right amount of food, if this level is additionally reduced by regular vomiting or low appetite feeling, it can lead to under-supply.

This also applies to naturally thin people who have a BMI below 20. For very thin people it would be fatal to lose even more health, which can happen due to a dietary ketogen. Also in this way serious deficiency symptoms can arise

- **The side effects**

With side effects is really only to be expected if pre-existing conditions or the abandonment of carbohydrates is too drastic. Therefore, it can come in the first phase of adaptation to side effects. The abrupt withdrawal of carbohydrates can lead to unwanted side effects. Common side effects include fatigue, bad breath, nausea, constipation, weakness, and muscle mass loss. This happens especially in the first few weeks of the diet change, as the body has to adapt to the new circumstances. The remedy here is to reduce the intake of carbohydrates step by step and to pay close attention to the physical reaction.

In order to minimize possible side effects, the omission of carbohydrates should not happen suddenly. More tolerable is a steady reduction in carbohydrates. As a result, while the entry of ketosis takes longer, but minimizes the chance of unwanted side effects. Also, it may come to relapses due to the sometimes severe side effects, which happens less often due to a longer-term adjustment of the carbohydrate amount.

High-performance athletes considering a ketogenic diet should painstakingly calculate their daily intake of nutrients, fats and carbohydrates and feed them to their bodies so that they can not be deficient. For intense sports that are run for a short time, the ketogenic diet is better than for fitness-oriented sports such as swimming or running. For the development of muscle mass, a ketogenic diet can support nutrition.

For vegans and vegetarians, the implementation of a ketogenic diet plan is quite difficult, because possibly meat, fish and animal products must be replaced by vegan and vegetarian products of equal value. It can sometimes be complicated to provide adequate nutrition on a vegetarian or vegetarian basis. Again, a well-designed nutrition plan can help.

Reasons You May Not Be Losing Weight On Keto Diet, Despite Your Best Efforts

Though keto diet is straightforward and easy to follow, however, sometimes this diet may not help you yield the desired results. Well, this may happen due to some of the following reasons:

1. You May be Gobbling Down Too Many Calories

The basic idea of this diet is to include more fats but sometimes people may pile up on so many fats without even checking on the calorific intake. It is equally important to keep your calorific intake under check, or else the diet won't work.

2. No Ketosis Happening

Your body needs to mend the metabolism and shift towards burning fats instead of carbohydrates, also known as ketosis. Sometimes, people may be blindly following the diet without keeping track of what they are consuming, which may hinder ketosis.

3. More Protein Intake

You may be on a low carbohydrate diet but if you are consuming more amounts of protein, that may also defeat the purpose of the diet. Remain within your dietary limits of consuming protein for the diet to work well.

4. More Carbohydrates

Including more than required amounts of carbohydrates can take you back from where you started or derail your entire efforts. Maintain your carbohydrate intake, or else you may not monitor any changes in your weight.

5. You May be Eating Less

Because of your dietary restriction or to be in sync with the diet, some people may reduce their calorie intake to extreme levels. Any kind of extremity may take a toll on the efficacy of the diet. Therefore, eating lesser calories than required may also affect your progress.

6. Any Kind of Food Allergies

If, while following this diet, you develop any kind of food allergies, it may spoil your progress. This is because food allergies or any kind of food intolerance increases the inflammation and inflammation may lead to weight gain.

7. If You Develop Leptin Resistance

Leptin is a hunger hormone, which helps in sending a signal to the brain when the body feels satiated. However, sometimes due to stress, lesser calorie intake, increased calorie intake or sleep issues, the functionality of this hormone may get affected leading to leptin resistance. If you become leptin resistant, your body is unable to send proper signals to the brain.

We hope that the keto diet helps you lose weight. If you have any queries in making major dietary choices, consult your dietician for the same.

Persevere the ketogenic diet

Especially the first days are often difficult for newcomers. As the body switches to the ketogenic diet, unpleasant side effects such as bad breath, tiredness, sleeping problems, and digestive problems are common. It may therefore make sense not to completely abstain from carbohydrates from the beginning. It is better to first switch to a low-carb diet such as the well-known Atkins diet and gradually cut off the carbohydrates from the diet.

✓ Pros: Benefits of the ketogenic diet
The ketogenic diet has several advantages:

- The fat deposits in the body melt quickly.

- Degrading the glucose stores leads to drainage and thus further weight loss.

- Insulin levels remain constantly low. Food cravings are avoided.

- Athletes like the ketogenic diet because dehydration helps better control the trained muscles and builds strength.

- Medicine has found that a ketogenic diet has a positive impact on certain diseases such as epilepsy. This is because the ketones also affect the metabolism of the brain, so it is less likely to epileptic seizures. In children who had been feeding ketogenically for two years, one study even found that their epilepsy was healing.

- Very helpful is the ketogenic diet in type 2 diabetes or prediabetes, as it has a direct influence on insulin levels. An American study found that 7 out of 21 participants were able to do without their diabetes medication after the change in diet.

- Researchers also have high hopes that a ketogenic diet can halt the progression of Alzheimer's disease. Studies have shown that an Alzheimer's brain can no longer use any sugar it needs as a source of energy. However, it can utilize ketone bodies and derive its energy from fat. Similar research is being done in oncology after initial experiments showed that the ketogenic diet could positively affect cancer.

✓ Cons: Disadvantages of the ketogenic diet

A ketogenic diet should in principle only be done for a limited period of time to attack the fat deposits. In the long run, the body can not function without carbs and sugar.

A novice mistake is choosing the wrong foods. Many people assume that a "high-fat diet" is a license to eat large quantities of greasy meat. In fact, protein-containing foods such as meat and fish should only be consumed in moderation. More important are high-quality vegetable fats such as olive oil and rapeseed oil, nuts and seeds, as well as the extremely healthy, high-fat avocado. This should include eggs, dairy products such as cottage cheese, fresh vegetables and fruit on the shopping list. A handful of walnuts, a hard-boiled egg or a bowl of olives are ideal snacks in the ketogenic diet

In order to avoid acidification of the body, a lot of water should be drunk between meals. The water flushes the acids out of the body.

What is ketosis?

Ketosis is a natural form of metabolism in which the body relies on fat for lack of carbohydrates and sugars to gain new energy. The liver transforms the fatty acids into so-called ketone bodies, which replace the usual glucose as "fuel". This process is called ketosis and has various health effects on the body.

Originally, ketosis was an emergency program of the body in times of famine and prolonged fasting. Because no carbohydrates and sugar were added to the body, the body uses fat deposits . However, in today's affluent society, carbohydrates and sugars are available to people all the time, everywhere. The fat deposits remain untouched or continue to grow, because the body is genetically programmed to provide for bad times. Only a ketogenic diet can bring it to ketosis today and melt the fat pads.

How the brain uses ketone bodies
The brain is the body's biggest "energy eater". When, in the middle of the day, the craving for something sweet awakens at work, usually the brain behind it, which calls for fresh energy in the form of sugar (glucose). However, the brain can also derive its energy from the ketone bodies that cross the blood-brain barrier. Already after three days of fasting, the brain gets about 25% of its energy from ketosis. However, because it does not get by without glucose, the brain sets the so-called gluconeogenesis in motion. In this metabolic process, the body transforms protein into glucose to feed the brain. In prolonged ketosis, the brain derives 70% of its energy from ketone bodies and 30% from gluconeogenesis.

Already in 1921, the ketogenic diet was first developed for the treatment of epilepsy in children. Although it has not yet been possible to clarify exactly which mechanisms are involved, studies have shown that half of the children involved were affected by epileptic seizures, and 15% were even spared attacks. Recent studies have shown similar promising results in the treatment of Alzheimer's, as well as in the treatment of other diseases such as Parkinson's and migraine.

Side effects of ketosis
In the first few days of ketosis, side effects such as gastrointestinal problems, increased need for sleep and typical fruity bad breath occur until the body gets used to the new diet and attacks the fat deposits. Most people then feel healthy and fit during the ketogenic diet.

When will I be in ketosis? The 10 most common ketosis signs

You've switched to the ketogenic diet so your body attacks the fat deposits to derive its energy. So you can effectively lose weight and improve your health. During the first few days of the ketogenic diet, your body must first switch. It produces less insulin and metabolizes the fat cells. This allows the liver to produce ketones and provide the brain with energy- The process of ketosis.However, it is difficult for newcomers to recognize whether your body is already in the ketosis or not. That's why you'll find 10 unmistakable ketosis signs that tell you you're already in ketosis.

Pay attention to these 10 ketosis signs:

1. Bad breath

Bad breath is an unmistakable sign of ketosis. Many people who start a ketogenic diet or follow a low-carbohydrate diet like Atkins find that their breath smells more fruity at one go. This is due to the elevated ketone levels, or more precisely, to acetone, a ketone that is found in the breath and urine. Bad breath is not pleasant, but you can help yourself with sugarless chewing gum and frequent brushing. After a while, the breath normalizes again

2. weight loss

A ketogenic diet like other low carb diets leads to effective weight loss. Especially in the first weeks, the pounds will melt quickly. However, these are not melting fat pads - the body now breaks down carbohydrates and water. When this process is over, you will lose weight slowly, but steadily, as long as you follow the diet.

3. More ketones in the blood

The ketogenic diet lowers blood sugar levels while increasing ketone levels. To determine if ketosis is already in full swing with you, you can use a special meter. This measures the level of beta-hydroxybutyrate (BHB) in the blood, one of the most important ketones. This should be between 0.5 and 3.0 mmol / l. Test strips (actually for diabetics) are available at the pharmacy or on the Internet.

4. More ketones in the breath or urine

The ketone level can be determined not only by the blood but also with a breath sample - another unavoidable ketosis indication. As already mentioned in point 1, the acetone level increases with progressive ketosis and causes bad breath. The acetone content can be checked with a special breath tester (Breathalyzer), but this method is considered less reliable than the blood sample. Alternatively, test strips are also a possibility for a urine sample.

5. loss of appetite

In ketosis, the body feels less appetite. Why this is so, the science could not yet clarify, but it is believed the filling diet with more protein and vegetables, and changes in hormone levels.

6. More energy and higher concentration

At the beginning of a ketogenic diet, many people feel tired, exhausted and mentally paralyzed. This condition is also known as "keto flu". Once this "flu" has been overcome and ketosis has occurred, the brain gets its energy from ketones instead of glucose. Ketones are a great source of energy, and in the longer term they even improve brain function. Medical studies have shown that ketones are effective in concussions and memory loss. Therefore, after the initial exhaustion, you feel highly concentrated and mentally energetic.

7. tiredness

As mentioned in point 6, keto flu often occurs during the transition. You feel tired and tired because your body takes awhile to adjust to the new energy source of ketones. During this time, it may be useful to support the body with additional electrolytes. These are lost to him through the drainage.

8. Less physical performance

Keto flu does not just affect the brain. The body also initially suffers from the changeover because it is no longer supplied with the familiar energy. During this time you may find that you can not bring the usual athletic achievements. But no worry. After a while, the body has changed and you feel the benefits of the ketogenic diet. So you will burn more fat while exercising. One study found that athletes with ketogenic nutrition burned up to 230% more fat than others.

9. Digestive problems

A major change in diet is initially difficult to manage for the gastrointestinal tract. The ketogenic diet makes no difference and you may be suffering from diarrhea or constipation. After a while, the change has taken place and the intestinal activity normalizes again. Make sure you eat as much fresh vegetables as possible: it contains few carbohydrates and provides you with important fiber.

10. Insomnia

The drastic reduction of carbohydrates leads to insomnia in many people. Again, this is (unfortunately) a typical ketosis indication. After a few weeks you should be able to sleep normally again. Some people who follow a ketogenic diet for longer sleep even better.

Doing Aerobic Exercise With a Ketogenic Diet

Many prefer doing an exercise that is done with a combination of body movements; just like the aerobic exercise with the cyclical ketogenic diet. It is not really an easy way to do because it requires a lot of energy in performing it. This kind of exercise is not advisable to those who are on a restricted calorie diet especially when their energy is also affected. When doing an aerobic exercise you must have enough energy to accomplish it but how will you able to do it if you are just eating a limited amount of food. Once an individual is on a diet he or she can only do limited activities. It can even make them easily get tired and become weak. This does not happen when you are on a ketogenic diet.

It doesn't mean that when you are already on a diet you will also become healthy. Actually, it is the most affected in your life because you are not eating enough food to give your body the nutrients that it needs. You may become slimmer but your health will be in great danger. The only thing that you can do is to invest into dietary supplements that aside from losing weight it will also provide your body with the nutrients that it requires. There are a lot of products that promises this kind of benefits but most of it does not give your body the right amount of energy to do intense task. With the ketogenic diet you will not just achieve the perfect body that you wish to have but you will also acquire huge amount of energy that you can use to do other job or the aerobic exercise.

Aerobic exercise with ketogenic diet is the perfect combination that you can ever encounter since most of us want to have a physically fit and healthy body. With these two factors you can achieve the body that you want and still have enough energy to so some exercise. Diet will always be useless if you will not do an exercise. Imagine yourself losing weight but not having a firm and fit body. This is what will most likely happen to you if you lack an exercise when you are having your diet. You may reduce weight but your body structure will not be in perfect shape.

There are hundreds of companies that promote effective weight loss products as well as programs. In order to purchase the right one you must compare each of these and know its difference. You can set factors that you will follow base from what you want in a dietary product or program. With this process it would be much easier for you to decide what brand you will purchase. However, in case you are haven't got any idea what to purchase why not choose s ketogenic diet. It has great benefits for anyone who will use it. With the combination of aerobic exercise with ketogenic diet you can be assured that you will not just be satisfied with the result but you will also be proud of it.

The 9 most important tips when starting a ketogenic diet for weightloss

General Overview

- Understand what keto is and what is not

Rather than relying solely on what a friend or co-worker told you about the keto diet, it's important to do your own research.

Here is a brief summary of what the ketogenic diet is:

The goal of a ketogenic diet is to achieve a metabolic state of ketosis.

Ketosis is a condition in which your body relies on fat to gain energy, including stored body fat, instead of glucose from carbohydrates.

To reach the state of ketosis, you need your net carbohydrates (total , less fiber) to up to 20-30 g per day and at the same time increase the intake of fat through the diet.

Despite what you may have heard, you do not have to eat fat exclusively at Keto. Keto is not (necessarily) a high-fat, high-protein diet such as the Atkins diet.

Instead, it's a very low-carbohydrate diet that does not necessarily limit protein or fat, although most keto lovers stick to the following macronutrient ratio:

- Nutrient distribution in the ketogenic diet

70-80% healthy fats , such as coconut oil , MCT oil, olive oil and avocados

20-25% protein from organic meat, eggs and wild caught fish

5-10% carbohydrates from low carbohydrate vegetables

If you are just starting a ketogenic diet, there is a keto tip that you should not skip: determining your individual carbohydrate needs based on your goals and level of activity.

• Calculate your macronutrient needs

One common mistake many keto beginners make is to follow the general guideline to eat 20 grams of carbs per day.

Such a strategy may work initially, but could eventually lead to unwanted side effects such as fatigue or overeating.

It may be that you need more or less carbohydrates to support your goals. A person who does a lot of sports or is very active in the daytime at work can eat more carbohydrates in Keto than a person who exercises a sedentary lifestyle.

Instead, you should identify your personal macronutrient needs to know the exact amount of fat, carbohydrates, and proteins your body needs to support your goals and lifestyle.

The easiest and most effective way to keep your target macaroons is to cook as many keto meals as possible.

:

Preparation and patience are the key when you first start keto - but before you go straight to the supermarket, there is another fundamental step to take.

- Determine your goal, your personal "why"

To get into ketosis requires commitment. So it's a good idea to sit down and find out about your commitment and why you want to try this new way to eat.

Do you want to have more energy with the ketogenic diet to play with your children? Or is it important to you to be able to concentrate better at work? Or do you want to successfully lose weight with keto and get your wish figure?

Or maybe you are finally ready to take your health into your own hands.

Instead of focusing on superficial goals like "lose 5 pounds", you should definitely find out the reason for the goal.

In this way, you can relate to your "why" and keep disciplined to your ketogenic diet, if you do not have a keto snack or the symptoms of keto-flu your life difficult.

Fortunately, there are 9 efficient keto tips that will help you make the transition to ketosis.

9 essential keto tips for beginners

The keto diet does not have to be complicated, but it may require some preparation.

Use the following basic keto tips and you'll be on your way to more energy, fat loss, mental clarity and all the health benefits of the low carb high fat diet.

1: Watch for hidden carbohydrates

Carbohydrates are everywhere.

From dressings to sauces and breaded meat - flours and carbohydrate-rich thickeners hide everywhere.

The best thing you can do when you first start keto is:

Always read the nutritional information and ingredient list: Do not assume that you know the amount of carbohydrates or that you can estimate them. Always check the ingredient list and nutritional information of a food. And if it is not labeled, such as pumpkin or a banana, google the name of the food + the carbohydrate content.

Ketosnacks in between: Find snacks with low carbohydrates and high-quality, nutrient-rich ingredients and keep them handy at any time of hunger.

Also, consider tracking your carbs: it helps a lot to track your food the first week and keep track of what you eat. So you get a sense of what foods contain how many carbohydrates and what meals you can eat to absorb no more than 20-50 grams of carbs per day.

Even a small amount of carbs can increase your blood sugar, increase your insulin levels and throw you out of the ketosis.

2: Drink a lot of water and electrolytes

When your body starts to go into ketosis, it will use up its glycogen stores.

This means that your body releases and "rinses out" stored glucose. You will then find that you have to go to the bathroom more often because your body has more water to excrete.

This diuretic effect is transient, but it increases the risk of dehydration during the first few weeks of a ketogenic diet. And with excessive urination, you also lose important electrolytes and minerals.

Loss of electrolyte and water can cause headache and muscle pain - two symptoms of keto-flu.

To avoid this, drink plenty of water as you go into the ketosis and replace lost electrolytes with a targeted mineral supplement or by adding sea salt to your water.

A very good way to balance the electrolyte and mineral loss is to drink bone broth during a ketogenic diet.

3: Make intermittent fasting

Many people use fasting or intermittent fasting (interval fasting) to get into ketosis faster.

Calorie restriction helps you burn your glycogen stores faster, which can result in a faster transition and fewer symptoms of ketograms.

Intermittent fasting is a great option for many people who do not want to do long-term fasting or for whom it is out of the question to give up food for a longer period of time.

Interval fasting lets you choose a fasting window of 8, 12 or 16 hours - and yes, sleep counts as part of fasting.

To start intermittent fasting, try fasting for 8-10 hours between dinner and breakfast the next day.

As your body adjusts, you can increase the fasting window to 12-18 hours.

4: Move more and do sports

Especially in the first week of a ketogenic diet you will probably experience some symptoms of keto flu such as headache , muscle pain or less energy.

Instead of crawling into your bed, try to overcome yourself and do sports or exercise.

Light movement can actually help in the transition to ketosis by helping you to burn glycogen stores quickly .

Exercises such as jogging, swimming, or yoga will get your blood moving without losing your energy.

And once you're completely into ketosis (after 2-3 weeks), you can increase your exercise intensity. You may even notice an improvement in your energy and exercise performance.

5: Do not eat "unhealthy" carbs

The ketogenic diet limits your carbohydrate intake quite dramatically.

But that does not mean that you should take your daily carbohydrate intake with just a single, sugary meal or piece of bread.

This is called "Dirty Keto". It refers to eating as much inferior food as you like, as long as you stick to its macronutrient ratios. But that's not such a good idea.

"Unhealthy" keto foods with carbohydrates are often made from processed meats and sausages and very few nutrient-rich foods.

While technically they are within the ketone guidelines and contain few carbohydrates, they are terrible for you and you should only enjoy them in small amounts, if at all.

This includes all processed foods such as sausages, salami, finished products, etc.

Instead choose nutrient-rich, natural foods that support your health and your body.

And while proper diet and exercise are important cornerstones of your keto journey, you will not reach your full keto potential if you do not keep these two next tips in mind.

6: Keep your stress level low

Too much stress and chronic stress affects the body at the biological level.

A high level of cortisone (the main stress hormone) can interfere with the production of sex hormones and has been shown to increase weight.

So as you make these adjustments to your diet and your level of activity, do not forget to focus on lowering your stress levels , both at home and at work.

Writing a journal, yoga and meditation are some simple and effortless ways to reduce stress in the long run.

These activities can also make sure that you follow this next tip as well.

7: Ensure enough restful sleep

A poor quality of sleep or lack of sleep can unbalance your hormones and make it harder for you to lose weight with keto and avoid food cravings .

Place great emphasis on an optimal evening routine for more and better sleep :

- Avoid all screens and artificial blue light for at least one hour before going to bed.

- Sleep in a completely dark room.

- Make sure your bedroom is cool - about 15-18 ° C degrees.

- Stick to fixed times at bedtime and getting up.

- Make sure you get at least 7 hours of sleep a night .

- Start implementing these simple changes, and you will not only get more sleep, but also better sleep quality.

- And that means less craving for sugar and more energy during the day.

8: Use MCT oil

You should seriously consider adding MCT oil to your ketogenic diet.

This is especially true if you need a *q*uick boost of energy in the morning. MCT Oil can be easily consumed with a Bulletproof Coffee or simply put in your black coffee.MCT oil is also an easy way to increase your ketone levels to help your body get into ketosis faster.

Many people report an increase in energy and mental clarity after taking MCT oil.

Ketones are also able to travel directly through the blood-brain barrier to reach your brain cells more quickly. This explains the improved mental clarity and increased thinking.

MCTs have been associated with weight loss:

- Overweight and obese people successfully lost weight in a diet containing many medium chain fatty acids (MCTs) .

- A high-MCT diet can significantly reduce body weight and fat, even more than a diet high in long-chain triglycerides .

- The successful weight loss is partly because MCTs help to reduce appetite.Stimulates metabolism

- A ketogenic diet paired with MCT oil can provide you with even more of the amazing health benefits of ketosis, as you can produce more ketones and thus get into ketosis faster.

9: Eat more fat

If you frequently crave carbohydrates or cravings for sweets during your conversion to keto, try adding more healthy fats to your diet.

MCT oil (medium chain triglycerides), coconut oil, macadamia nut and avocado fatty acids help quench cravings and balance blood sugar levels .

You can take care of calorie restriction and meal tracking later.

When you pass into ketosis, the main goal is to stick to keto-friendly prescriptions, keep carbohydrates low, and survive the first few weeks without too many ketograms.

Losing weight with the ketogenic diet - The 7-day nutrition plan for you

Here is a nutrition plan for the one-week ketogenic diet:

- ✓ **Sunday**
- ✓ Breakfast: poached egg with avocado

- ✓ Lunch: Salad of your choice with tuna fillet

- ✓ Evening: Wraps - instead of a wheat tortilla you use a sushi kelp leaf to wrap around

- ✓ Snack: Chips of kale

- ✓ **Monday**
- Breakfast: kale smoothie, cucumber, celery and apple wedges

- At lunchtime: zucchini pasta with tofu, avocado and almond yoghurt (crush half a soft avocado with a fork and stir in 2 tablespoons of almond yoghurt)

- Evening: chicken soup

- Snack: 10 grams of almonds

✓ **Tuesday**
- Breakfast: scrambled egg of 2 eggs, 30 grams of avocado and 1 tomato

- Lunch : Bolognese made from beef tartare with konjag noodles

- In the evening: Grilled salmon with lettuce

- Snack: Apple slice with 2 spoons of peanut butter

✓ **Wednesday**
- Breakfast: Green smoothie from green vegetables

- Lunch: Large salad with roasted pumpkin and Tahin

- Evening: Garlic fried chicken and spinach

- Snack: A handful of sunflower seeds

✓ **Thursday**
- Breakfast: omelette with vegetables

- Lunch: salad of tuna, feta and cucumber

- Evening: turkey steak with green salad

- Snack: fried zucchini slices

✓ **Friday**
- Breakfast: Savory muffins made from egg, pepper and zucchini

- Lunch : Strips of beef fillet with salad

- In the evening: miso chicken soup

- Snack: hummus with cucumber for dipping

Saturday
- Breakfast: Veggie Frittata

- Lunch: broccoli soup

- Evening: lemon chicken with cauliflower rice and peanut dressing

- Snack: 3 apple slices with Tahin

Ketoegeni Diet Recipes For Weightloss

1. 4 Best Recipes for Low Carb Omelettes

Egg dishes such as omelettes are perfect for a low carb diet. They shine through an ultimate low carbohydrate content and since they can vary and refine their mood, omelets are not boring so soon at low carb. The important thing about the omelette is the consistency: it should be loose and nicely fluffy. Just chill the low carb omelette over medium heat and pull through the omelette with a fork. It will be nice and fluffy.

- **Leek ham omelette**

This low carb omelette recipe with the combination of leek and ham is simply terrific and ultimately satisfying. This keeps the three meals a day without any problems. Golden yellow and wonderful juicy.Perfect for breakfast.

- SERVINGS: 2 SERVINGS

INGREDIENTS:

- 200 g ham cooked

- 1 stick of leek

- 100 ml creme fraiche

- 50 ml of cream

- 50 g of Parmesan

- 3 eggs

- 2 egg yolks

- butter

- nutmeg

- salt

- pepper

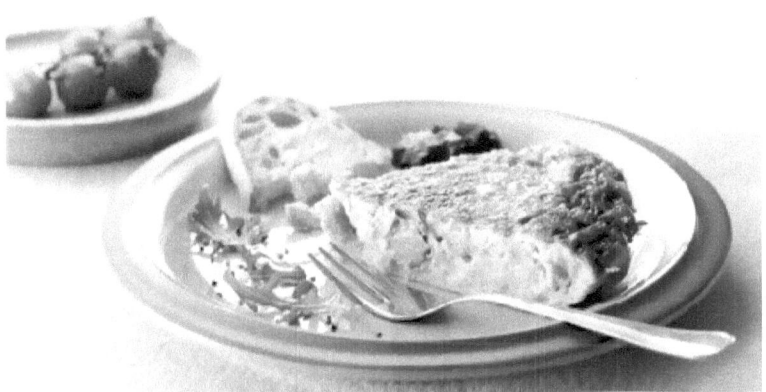

INSTRUCTIONS:

- Cut the leek lengthwise and cut into thin slices, dice the cooked ham.

- Put both in a buttered (not too big) pan and sauté. Put aside.

- Now boil the cream with the crème fraiche and stir in about 2/3 of the parmesan, so that it slowly melts.

- Then remove from the heat, add the eggs and egg yolk, mix to a homogeneous mass and season with salt, pepper and nutmeg.

- Meanwhile preheat the oven to 160 degrees.

- The mass consisting of eggs, cream, creme fraiche now over ham and leeks and sprinkle the remaining Parmesan over the omelet.

- Now cook the omelette in the oven for about 20 minutes.

- **Spinach omelette**

The mix makes it! In this recipe it's the mix of spinach, spring onion and fresh basil. Incidentally, this low carb omelette also tastes great with some feta.

- SERVINGS: 2 SERVINGS

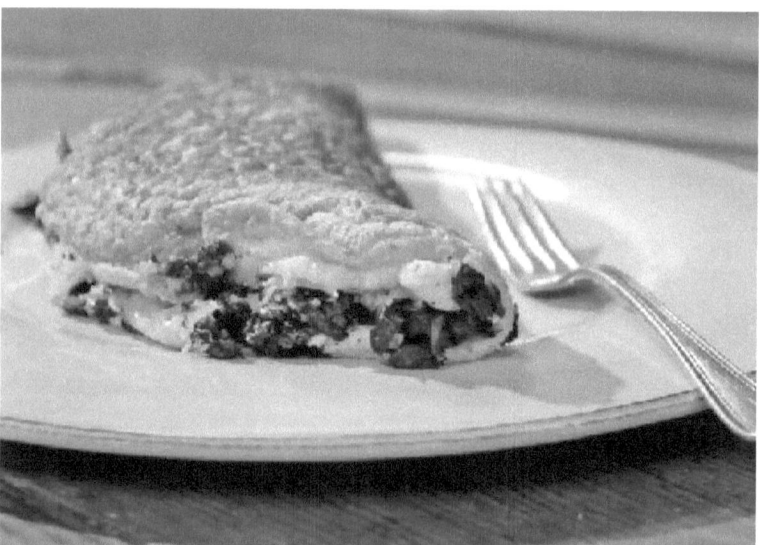

INGREDIENTS:

- 3 hands full of leaf spinach

- 3 spring onions
- 8 leaves of basil
- 3 eggs
- milk
- 1/2 onion
- 3 cherry tomatoes
- 2 tbsp oil
- Some garlic
- nutmeg
- salt
- pepper

INSTRUCTIONS:

- Clean spring onions and cut into fine rings. Now fry with the finely chopped onion and garlic in a pan. Then add the tomatoes and spinach.
- In the meantime whisk the eggs with the milk and season with salt, pepper and nutmeg.
- Once the spinach has collapsed in the pan, pass the egg mass over it.
- Now let the omelette falter over medium heat.
- Turn over after about 4 to 5 minutes, so that it takes on the other side of a gold-brown color.

- **Broccoli cheese omelet**

Whether as a breakfast, lunch or dinner - this delicious low carb omelette always tastes great! The broccoli with its high content of minerals, vitamins and trace elements ensures that we eat healthy and balanced. By the way, this omelet is super filling too!

- SERVINGS: 1

INGREDIENTS:

- Cooked about a handful of broccoli florets
- 1 egg
- 2 egg whites
- 1 tbsp milk
- 1-2 tablespoons of grated cheese
- Some oil
- salt
- pepper

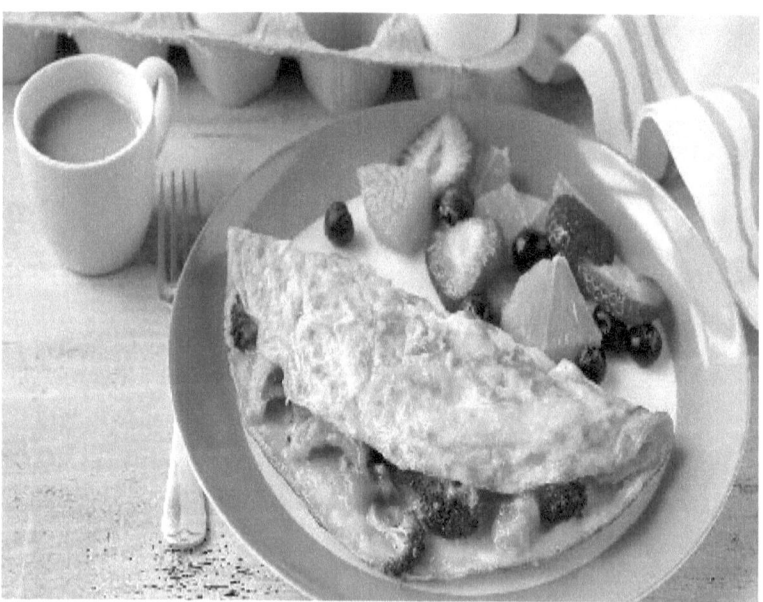

- Whisk the egg together with the egg whites and milk, salt and pepper.

- Heat some oil in a pan and add the egg and milk mixture to the pan. Reduce heat.

- Now sprinkle the cheese over the slowly solidifying mass and place the broccoli florets in the middle.

- **Omelette rolls with salmon and cream cheese**

If you are looking for a refined Low Carb Omelette that is great as a small but delicious low carb appetizer, then Omelette Rolls are sure to be the right choice.

- SERVINGS: 12 ROLLS

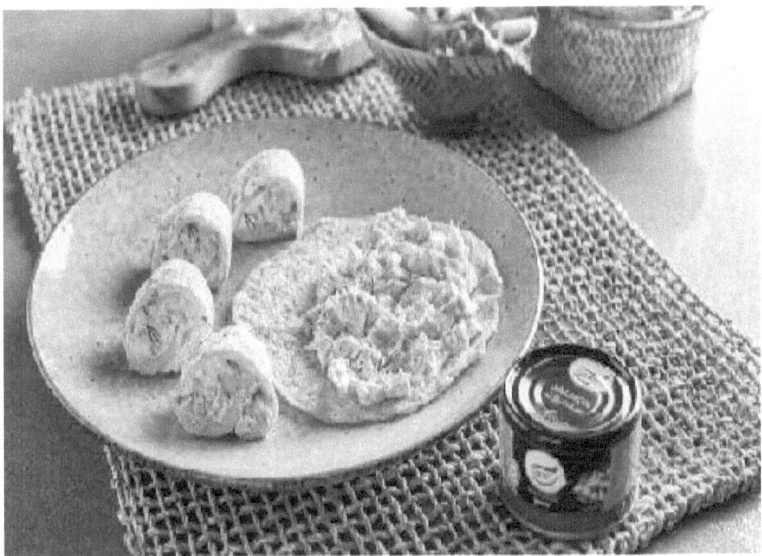

INGREDIENTS:

- 8 eggs

- 8 tbsp mineral water

- Smoked 200 g salmon

- 200 g cream cheese

- rapeseed oil

- Some rocket

- salt

- pepper

- Wooden skewer / Party skewers

INSTRUCTIONS:

- Whisk eggs, mineral water, salt and pepper

- Heat some rapeseed oil in a non-stick pan (about 20 cm) and add a quarter of the egg mixture to the pan

- Stir at medium heat until the omelet is firm on top, turn over and fry for another 2 minutes from the other side

- Remove and bake three more omelets and let cool

- Spread the omelets with cream cheese, cover with rocket and smoked salmon and roll up

- Cut into three slanted pieces and fix with skewers

- Ready to serve.

2. Low carb pancakes

Pancakes are very popular with young and old. Especially because they are prepared so fast, can be varied in variety and of course because they are so incredibly delicious.

- SERVINGS: 2 PEOPLE

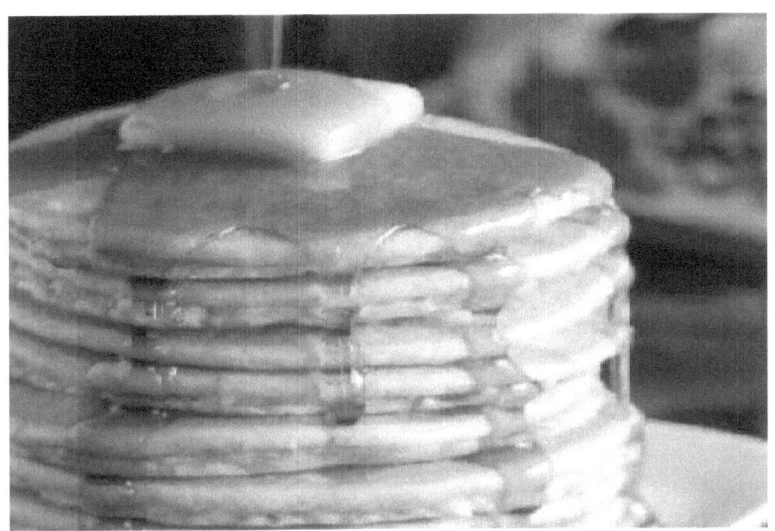

INGREDIENTS:

- 100 ml soymilk
- 3 egg whites
- 50 g soy flour or almond flour
- 2 pinches of salt
- 0.5 teaspoon baking powder
- Sweet

UPON NEED:

- cinnamon
- Fresh fruits

INSTRUCTIONS:

- Beat the three egg whites into a firm egg whites. Put aside
- Now add the soy milk together with the soy or almond flour, the baking powder and the salt in a mixing bowl and mix everything to a smooth mass.
- Now sweeten the dough as you like and then lift it very carefully under the egg whites.
- Now the dough comes in portions in a coated pan.

3. Low carb recipe for egg whites
- SERVINGS : 8 EGG WHITES

INGREDIENTS:

- 140 ml of water
- 100 g of lean quark
- 75 g protein powder, neutral
- 3 tablespoons chia seeds
- 2 tablespoons psyllium husk
- 0.5 sachet of baking powder
- 1.5 teaspoons salt
- 1 egg
- 4 tbsp topping (sesame, poppy seeds, sunflower seeds, pumpkin seeds)

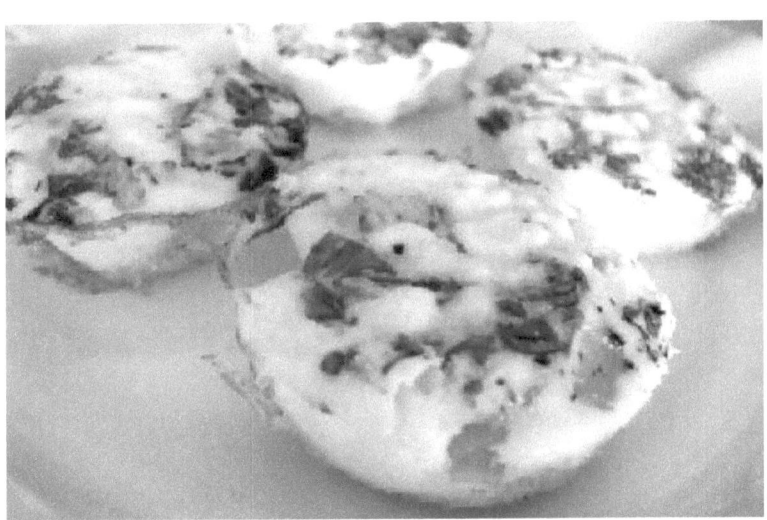

INSTRUCTIONS:

- Place the protein powder, chia seed, psyllium husk, baking powder and salt in a mixing bowl and mix together

- In a second mixing bowl, mix the curd cheese, the egg and the water into a creamy mixture

- Now combine the contents of both mixing bowls and stir into a dough, let rest for 10 minutes

- Preheat the oven to 180 ° C (hot air)

- Lay out a baking sheet with parchment paper

- Now sprinkle the seeds and seeds on a plate and mix briefly

- Divide the dough into 8 equal pieces. Roll each piece into a ball and then toss briefly on the prepared plate with the seeds and seeds

- Place the egg whites on the baking paper and let them brown in the oven for 15 to 17 minutes

4. Low carb recipe for baked Camembert

The Camembert is very well suited for the low-carb dinner. The baked Camembert is either a solo or with cranberries or a delicious salad.

SERVINGS: 2 PEOPLE CALORIES: 312 KCAL

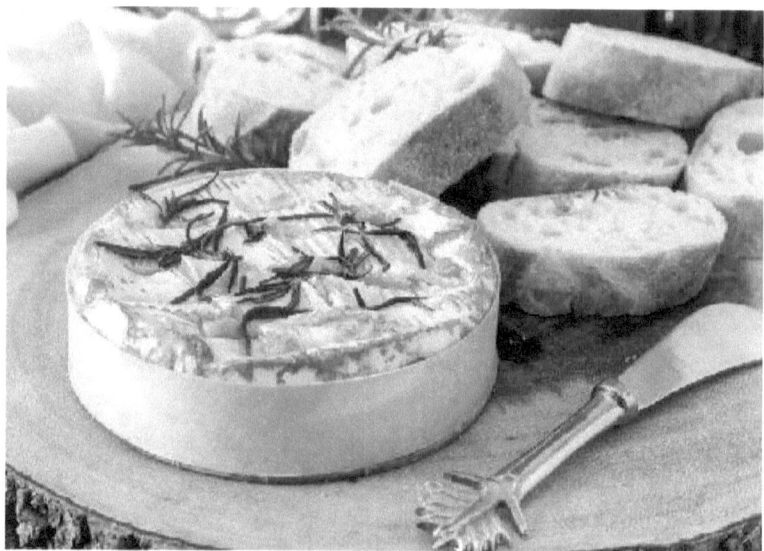

INGREDIENTS:

- 2 Camemberts
- 1 egg
- Some breadcrumbs

- A little rapeseed oil
- Some butter

INSTRUCTIONS:

- Put the egg in a deep plate and whisk it lightly
- Place the breadcrumbs and the oil in another deep plate
- Now turn the Camemberts first in oil, then in the egg and finally in the breadcrumbs
- Cover in hot butter in a non-stick pan over low heat and fry for about 10 minutes, turning it from side to side over several times
- If the Camembert rises a little, it is good, the cheese is then melted inside

5. Low carb recipe for green roast peppers with sea salt

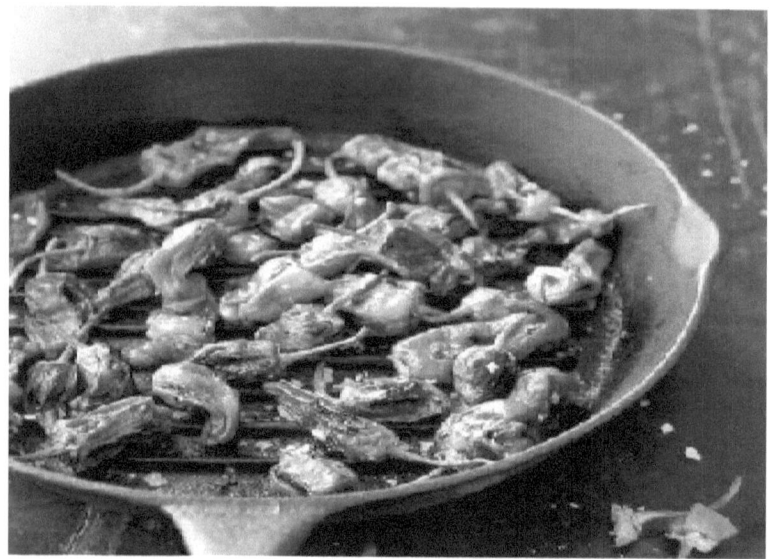

If you've ever been to Spain in a typical tapas bar, you've probably seen them be-fore, green roast peppers traditionally served with sea salt and better known in Spain . This recipe does not need much. Just a few fried peppers , some sea salt and olive oil.

SERVINGS: 2 PEOPLE , CALORIES: 14 KCAL

INGREDIENTS:

- 200 g of green pepper green

- sea-salt

- olive oil

INSTRUCTIONS:

- Clean the fried peppers

- Heat the olive oil in a pan and roast the peppers all around until the skin throws bubbles
- Serve on a plate, sprinkle with sea salt and serve immediately

6. Gluten-free low carb bread

For those who do not have gluten and are low in carbohydrates, finding bread that meets both needs is not that easy. But here is the solution: A gluten-free low-carb bread or alternatively gluten-free low-carb bread rolls. Its recommended keeping the bread in a freezer bag in the refrigerator from the 3rd day onwards. You can personally toast the bread slices a bit. But that's a matter of taste, as you know.

- SERVINGS: 12 SLICES

INGREDIENTS:

- 180 ml of water boiling
- 80 g almonds ground, blanched
- 40 g of flaxseed flour neutral
- 40 g psyllium husk milled
- 30 g of hemp flour
- 30 g sunflower seeds
- 15 g of baking powder
- 15 ml balsamic vinegar
- 2 eggs
- 1 egg white
- 2 tablespoons sesame, pumpkin seeds, flaxseed
- 0.5 teaspoon sea salt

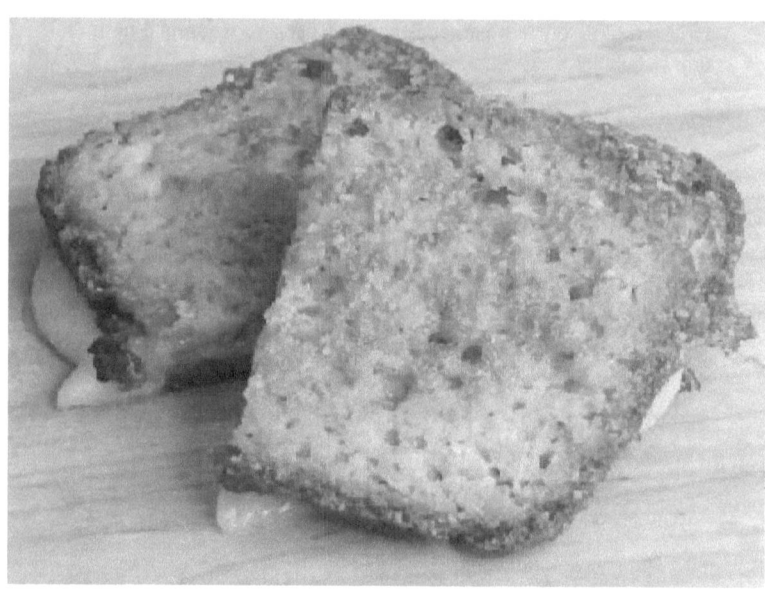

INSTRUCTIONS:

- Put the ground almonds, hemp flour, flaxseed flour, psyllium husks, sun-flower seeds, salt and baking powder in a bowl and mix well

- Add the balsamic vinegar to the dry ingredients while stirring, then add the eggs and egg whites

- Boil the water and add it to the dough while stirring to make a uniform dough

- Now preheat the oven to 180 ° C, remove a baking sheet from the oven and lay out with baking paper

- Put the bread dough on the baking sheet and shape into a flat, longish bread

- Sprinkle with sesame seeds, pumpkin seeds, sunflower seeds or flaxseed as needed, lightly press

- Put the bread in the oven for 70 minutes (top / bottom heat)

- After the baking time has elapsed, switch off the oven and turn the bread over and leave it in the oven for another 5 minutes

- Turn the bread over again and leave it in the oven with the oven door slightly open for another 5 minutes. This ensures that the bread does not collapse

7. low carb pancakes without flour

Loose-light pancakes are perfect for Sunday breakfast. So you can start in peace and with a lot of enjoyment in the day off. That pancakes without flour and without sugar can taste very delicious.

INGREDIENTS:

- 4 eggs

- 40 g protein powder neutral or vanilla flavor

- 2 tablespoons cream

- 1 banana

- Some butter

- Sweetness as needed

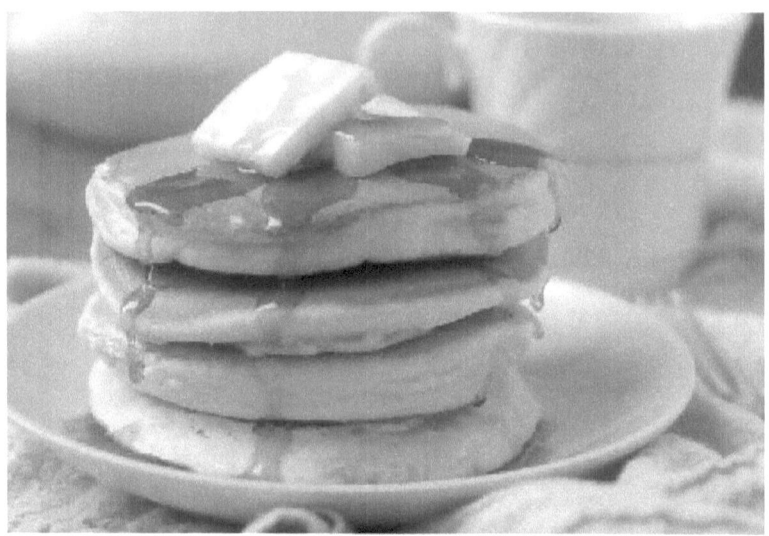

INSTRUCTIONS:

- Crush the banana with a fork, alternatively pour into the blender
- Now mix all ingredients to a creamy mass
- Heat the butter in the pan and add the pancake batter portion by portion into the pan.

8. low carb cheese chips

These cheese chips are ideal low-carb snacks and are prepared in no less than 5 minutes. Perfect for a small appetite in between or if it is necessarily something to nibble in front of the TV. A prerequisite for the success of the low carb cheese chips is that you still have some cheese in the fridge and that a microwave is within your reach.

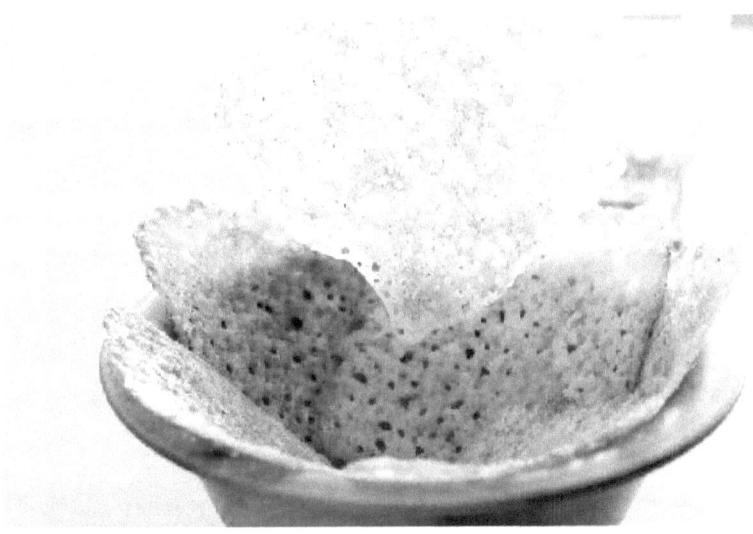

INGREDIENTS:

- Cheese Maasdamer, Gouda, everything the fridge gives

INSTRUCTIONS:

- Cut the cheese into bite-sized pieces or slices.
- Cut a baking paper so that it fits in the microwave.
- Now place the cheese pieces on the baking paper. Here, care should be taken to ensure that there is still enough space between the individual pieces of cheese, because the cheese - depending on the fat content - runs.
- Sizzling for about 4 minutes in the microwave at 800 watts.
- The cheese chips can be easily stored for 1 to 2 weeks in fresh food containers, so they are also ideal for traveling or for the office.

Tip: Of course you can also use cookie cutters to cut out stars, hearts, etc. from the cheese. Not only fun, but also looks really good!

9. Low carb almond milk

Almond milk is a popular drink, especially in southern Italy and Mallorca. Almonds are incredibly healthy because they strengthen the intestinal flora, lower the cholesterol level and provide the body important trace elements and minerals. And best of all, almond milk is not just low carb, it can also be refined to taste with a variety of ingredients. Vanilla extract, cinnamon, nutmeg, cocoa powder or a pinch of salt are especially suitable.

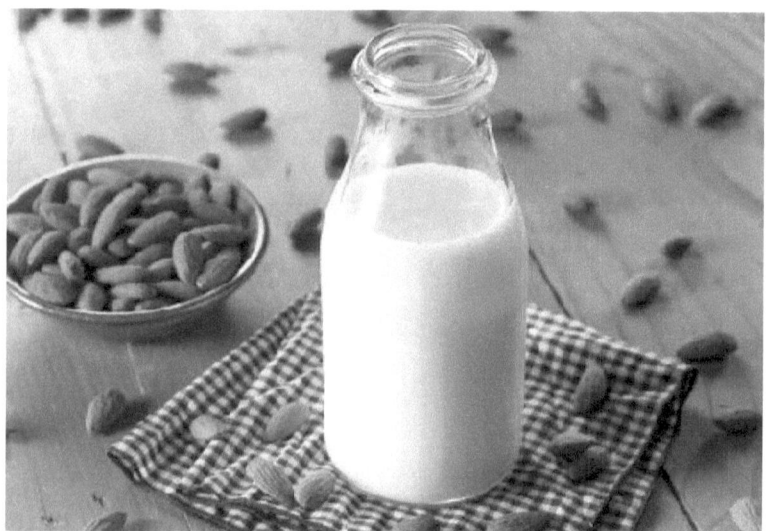

INGREDIENTS:

- 100 g blanched almonds

- 750 ml of water

- Stevia as needed

- 1 pinch of salt

INSTRUCTIONS

- A condition for the almond milk is a good blender. Add the almond in blender

- Gradually add the water until a milky liquid is formed. Now squeeze the liquid through a kitchen towel. Finally, season with stevia and a little salt.

- For those in a hurry: Almond mousse or purée is a little faster and easier. For this, add 2-4 tablespoons of almond purée to one liter of water and mix well.

10.low carb marble cake

This marble cake is a low carb dream - whether for breakfast or as dessert .

- SERVINGS: 12 PIECES

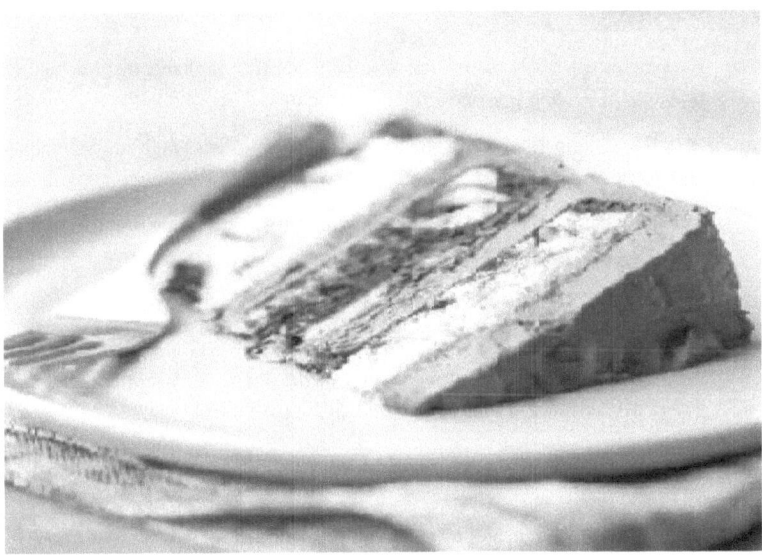

INGREDIENTS:

- 230 g almond flour

- 5 eggs

- 80 g butter soft

- 1 vial of butter-vanilla flavor

- 1 packet of baking soda

- 4 tbsp protein powder neutral

- 4 tablespoons of mascarpone

- 3 TL cocoa powder de-oiled

- Mineral water

- Sweetness to taste

INSTRUCTIONS:

- Beat the butter until creamy and gradually add the vanilla flavor, the baking powder, the protein powder and the mascarpone.

- Add the almond flour alternately with the eggs to the dough until finally a creamy mass is produced.

- Then sweeten to taste and add some mineral water depending on the consistency of the dough

- Now take about half of the dough and put it in a greased (and best with breadcrumbs swung out form) Gugelhupf form.

- Add the cocoa powder to the other half of the dough, stir well. If necessary, sweeten again.

- Now add the dark, cocoa-based mass to the light mass and use a fork to pull an "8" through the dough to create a light pattern.

- In the meantime preheat the oven to 160 ° C (hot air) and off with the marble cake for about 35 to 45 minutes in the oven.

- Its done and ready.

11. low carb bread rolls

Who says that you have to do without bread at Low Carb ? With a bit of creativity, you can quickly make some delicious low-carb bread rolls that have as many as 2.5 carbohydrates per roll. Sounds good? It is! Just try it!

- SERVINGS: 11 ROLLS

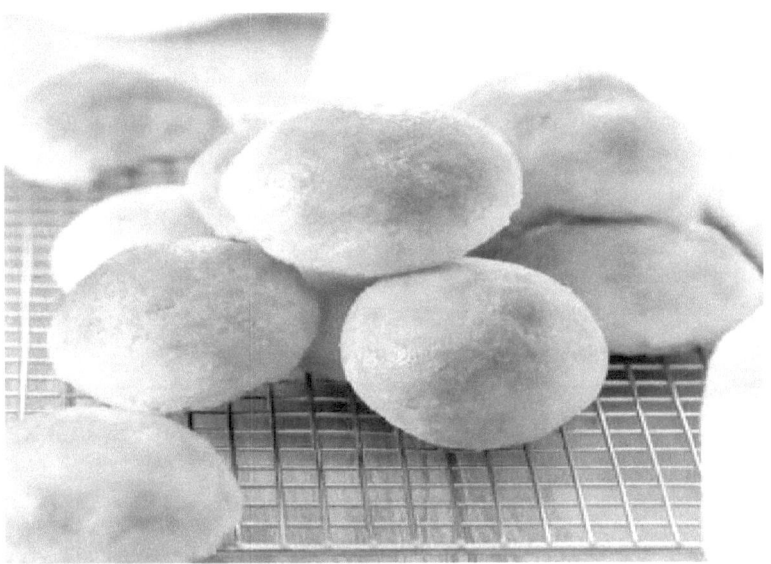

INGREDIENTS:

- 170 g of flaxseed ground

- 140 g of gluten

- 60 g almond flour

- 50 g pumpkin seeds

- 20 g sunflower seeds roughly chopped

- 10 g dry yeast

- 2 teaspoons salt
- 1 teaspoon bread spice
- 330 ml of lukewarm water
- Depending on your taste sesame caraway, poppy seeds

INSTRUCTIONS:

- Mix together Flaxseed, gluten, yeast, almond flour, salt and bread .
- Then gradually add the lukewarm water and knead for about 10 minutes to a consistent mass.
- Add pumpkin seeds and sunflower seeds and knead again.
- Now form the dough into rolls and place on a baking sheet lined with baking paper. Press flat and sprinkle with cumin, sesame seeds, poppy seeds or a mixture of grains to taste.
- Cover the rolls for about 45 minutes in a warm place.
- Then bake in the oven for 30 minutes at 180 ° C.

12.cheese bacon zucchini

Whether prepared on the grill or in the oven - the cheese-bacon-zucchini makes - not only at low carb - pretty good. And the preparation time takes only a few minutes.

- TIME: 40 MINUTES
- SERVINGS: 4 PEOPLE

INGREDIENTS:

- 4 about the same size zucchini
- 170 g breakfast bacon

- 140 g cheddar cheese

- 3 teaspoons olive oil

- salt

- pepper

INSTRUCTIONS:

- Preheat the oven to 180 ° C.

- Wash the zucchini, cut off the ends.

- Cut into the zucchini at intervals of about 1cm. Make sure that you do not cut through to the bottom.

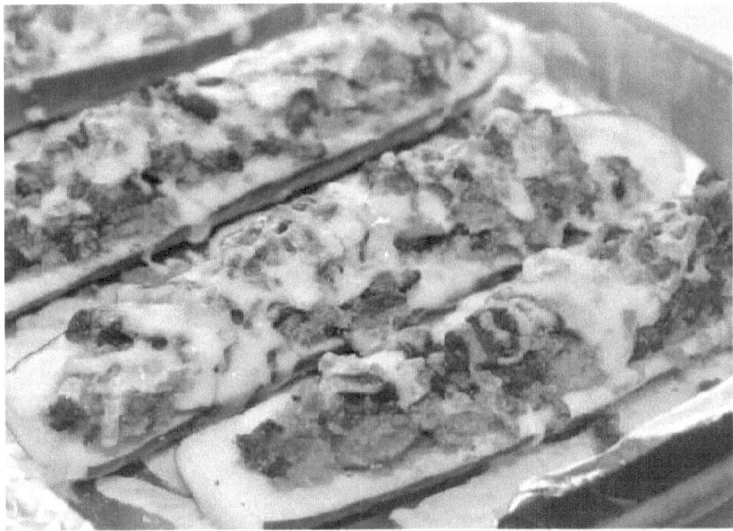

- Brush the slices with the olive oil, salt and pepper and then put in the oven at 180 ° C for about 15 minutes or put on the grill.

- In the meantime, cut the cheddar into bite-sized pieces.

- Fry the bacon crispy on both sides, place on a paper towel to cool and, when the bacon has cooled slightly, break into bite-sized pieces.

- At the end of the baking time, remove the courgettes from the oven or grill and fill the courgette loops with a piece of bacon and a piece of cheese.

- Put in the oven or on the grill for another 3 to 5 minutes until the cheese has run nicely.

- Its done and ready

13. Low carb recipe for a trout cream

The trout belongs to the family of salmon fish . In low carb ,trout plays a big role mainly because of the high quality and easily digestible protein content. Whether grilled, smoked, fried or just as a delicious trout cream for dipping - the trout is versatile in the kitchen.

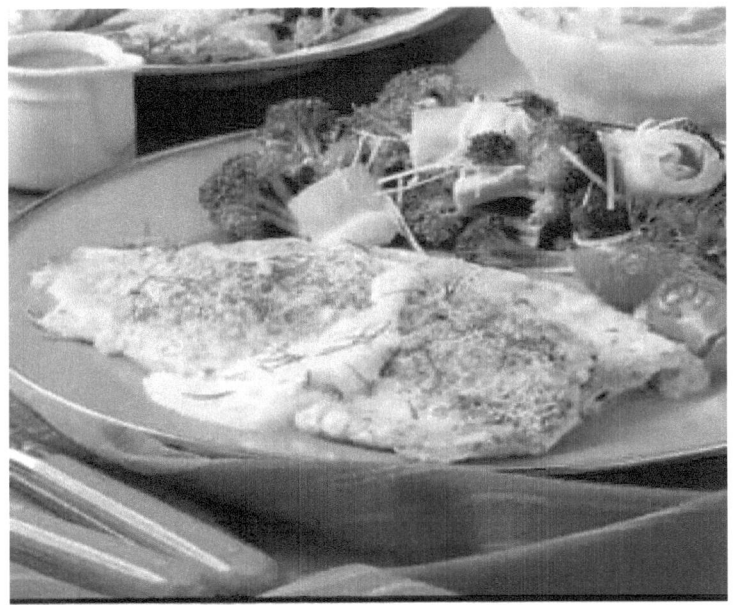

- SERVINGS: 2 PEOPLE

INGREDIENTS:

- 125 g trout fillets smoked
- 3 tablespoons remoulade or mayonnaise
- 3 tablespoons crème fraîche or cream cheese with or without herbs
- 1 Tomato chopped small, without pulp, so that the cream does not get too watery
- 1 teaspoon of flaxseed whole or broken
- 1 shot of lemon juice
- Possibly. a bit of chopped parsley or chives

- Pepper and salt to taste

- Crush the trout fillets with a fork, then add the remaining ingredients and stir well .

- For a change, you can also prepare this dip or spread very well with Stremel salmon, smoked mackerel or canned tuna. In that case please omit the lemon juice! For salmon fresh dill, mackerel or tuna, some very finely chopped onions and / or a dash of Worcester sauce.

14. Bacon egg muffins

Sunday mornings and you're fed up with omelets or scrambled eggs? No problem! Just get the muffin out of the cupboard and off you go. Because this recipe for delicious low carb bacon egg muffins is not only convincing because it's super easy, but also because the bacon is so deliciously crispy and the bacon egg muffins look great.

- SERVINGS: 6 MUFFINS

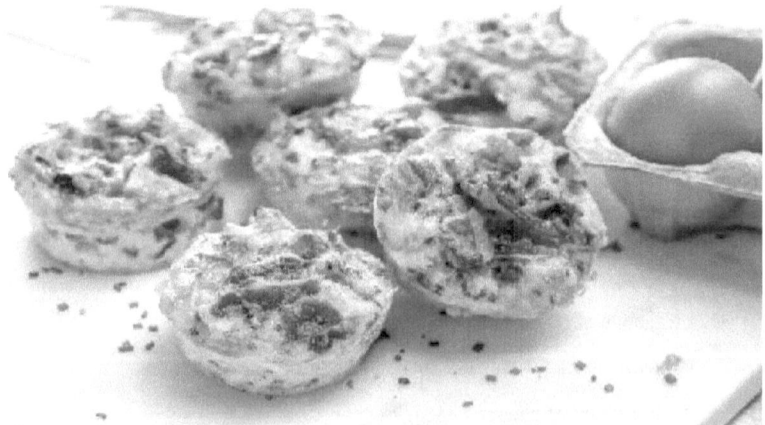

INGREDIENTS:

- 6 eggs
- 24 slices of bacon
- A little olive oil
- salt
- pepper
- Depending on the taste of some grated cheese

INSTRUCTIONS:

- Fry the bacon briefly in the pan so that it is crispy on all sides at the end. Meanwhile, you can Preheat the oven to 180 ° C.
- Grease the muffin dish with a little oil and slice each of the muffin shapes with four strips of bacon.
- Now add the egg, lightly salt and pepper (and, depending on your taste, sprinkle with some grated cheese) and bake in the oven for about 10 minutes.

15.crispbread

If you think that you have to do without crispbread at Low Carb, that's wrong! A great recipe that has come from the low carb community. Tastes great, is deliciously crunchy and satisfies very well, without making you tired. A slice of crispbread comes on just 3.8 grams of carbs.

- SERVINGS: 10 SLICES

INGREDIENTS:

- 150 g sunflower and pumpkin seeds
- 150 g of sesame seeds

- 100 g of chia seeds
- 3 eggs
- 100 ml of water
- salt

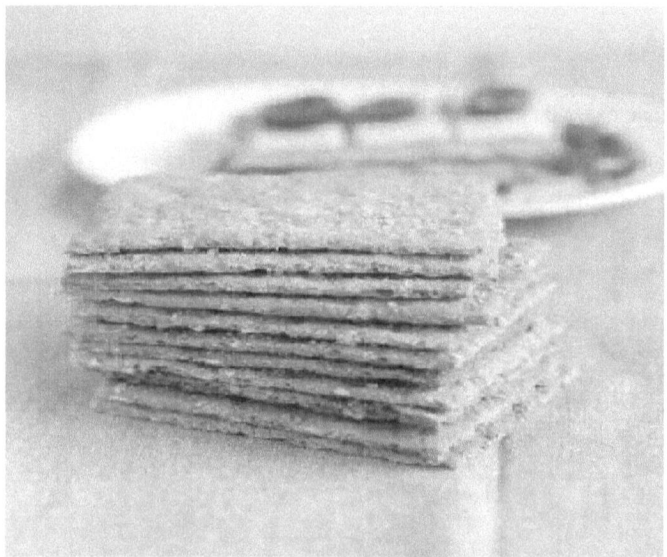

INSTRUCTIONS:

- Combine sunflower and pumpkin seeds as well as sesame seeds and chia seeds ,chop them up!
- Add eggs and 100ml of water and a pinch of salt and stir
- Spread the mixture on a baking sheet with baking paper, cut into strips with a knife and bake for 75 minutes in a convection oven 150 degrees.

16. Grilled asparagus

The beauty of asparagus is that you can use it so versatile. Whether white or green, in the oven, on the stove or on the grill - the possibilities are definitely diverse. For grilling green asparagus is usually better, because it is thinner than the white asparagus and thus faster is oven. Covered with a little olive oil, wrapped in bacon and topped off with sea salt, you get a delicious low carb side dish to the juicy steak in no time .

- SERVINGS: 2 PEOPLE

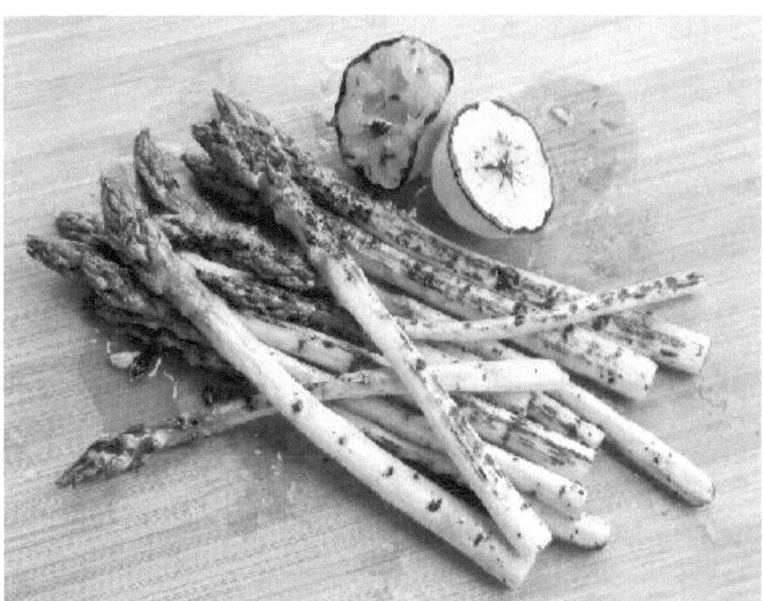

INGREDIENTS:

- 10 bars of asparagus green
- 10 slices of bacon

- olive oil

- sea-salt

- pepper

INSTRUCTIONS:

- First, remove the woody ends of the asparagus.

- Now brush with a little olive oil, salt, pepper and then wrap each with a slice of breakfast bacon.

- Approximately Grill and enjoy for 10 minutes over medium heat.

17.pumpkin muffins

As autumn approaches, and as it gets colder outside, the pumpkin season is breaking. But who thinks that one can only conjure pumpkin or pumpkin soup from the healthy saddlery is wrong. Here's a great low carb recipe for juicy pumpkin muffins .

- SERVINGS: 24

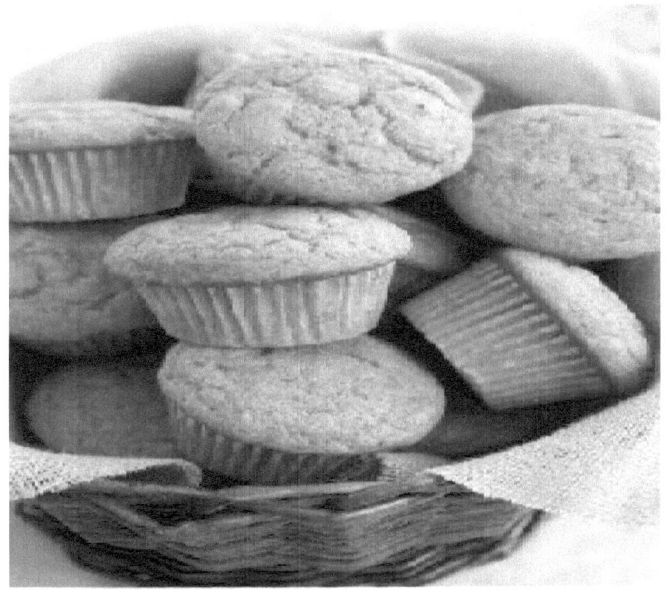

INGREDIENTS:

- 300 g almond flour
- 200 g of pumpkin puree
- 60 g of flaxseed flour
- 50 g butter soft
- Sweet
- 2 tsp pumpkin spice mixture
- 2 eggs
- 1 tsp vanilla extract
- 1 teaspoon soda

- 0.5 teaspoon baking powder

- 1 pinch of salt

- Refine walnuts or almond pieces with pecans as desired

INSTRUCTIONS:

- Preheat the oven to 180 ° C.

- Put the almond flour, flaxseed flour, baking powder, soda, salt and pumpkin spice in a mixing bowl.

- In a second bowl mix the butter, the pumpkin puree and the sweetness.

- Then add the eggs and the vanilla extract.

- Gradually add the ingredients of the first bowl to the egg and pumpkin mixture and stir until a smooth mass is formed.

- Now put the dough in muffin tin and bake for about 15 to 20 minutes until the muffins have a light golden-brown note.

18.peanut butter cookies

This low-carb biscuit recipe is perfect for days when you have cravings for sweets . These peanut butter cookies do not (almost) have to have a guilty conscience because after all they shine with their low carbohydrate content of just 1.1 g per biscuit and are therefore perfect for low carb .

- SERVINGS: 10 -11 BISCUITS

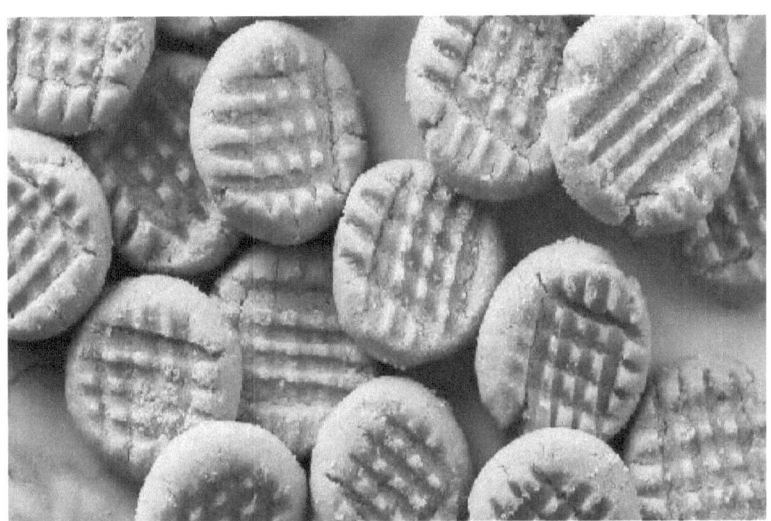

INGREDIENTS:

- 120 g peanut butter
- 1 egg
- 1 tsp vanilla flavor
- Sweetness to taste

INSTRUCTIONS:

- Knead all ingredients in a mixing bowl to a dough.
- use two teaspoons to form small balls and place them on a baking sheet lined with baking paper.
- Bake at 180 ° C for about 12 minutes until golden brown.
- Ready the peanut butter cookies!

19.low-carb crepes

Crepe - this is a form of egg cake that is especially popular in France. Whether sweet or spicy, the crepe has no limits in terms of taste. And since there are so many different variations with a little imagination and you will not get bored that fast.

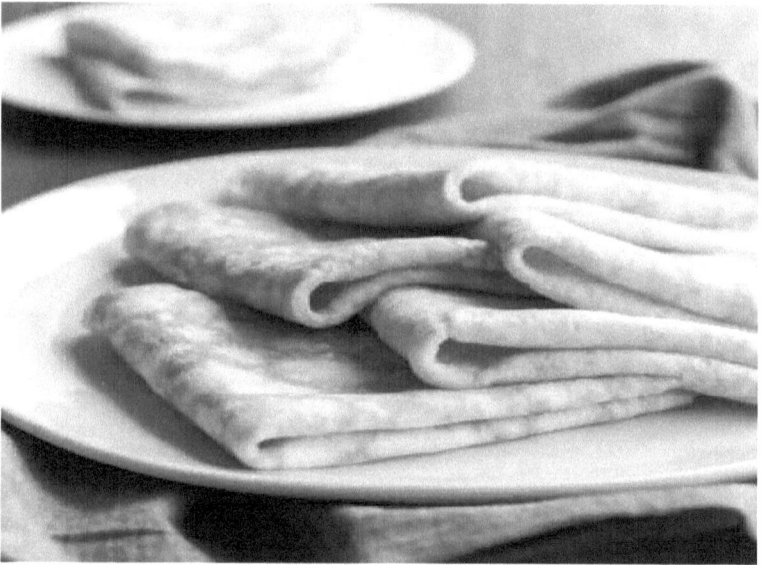

- SERVINGS: 9 CREPES

INGREDIENTS:

- 6 eggs
- 50 g of neutral protein powder
- about 20 g of peanut oil
- Some water

Those who prefer sweet crepes should let off steam on the following ingredients:

- Sweetness like xylith or erythritol
- Peanut butter
- Mandelmus
- cream cheese
- marzipan flavor
- Berry Mix
- Syrup without carbohydrates

For those who like it heartily:

- cheese
- sea-salt
- pepper
- paprika
- mushrooms
- Boiled ham
- cream cheese
- cottage cheese

INSTRUCTIONS:

- Mix the eggs with the protein powder to a creamy dough (add enough water to the dough to form a dough that will spread well in the pan).
- Now put some oil in the pan and distribute with a paper kitchen roll.
- Put about 2 tablespoons of dough in the pan, let it turn golden brown and turn it over.

20.Low carb recipe for chia pudding

Chia pudding in combination with goji berries - Superfood in a double pack! Superfood is a name given to naturally occurring foods that have a positive effect on our health through high levels of vitamins, minerals, antioxidants and vital essential amino acids.

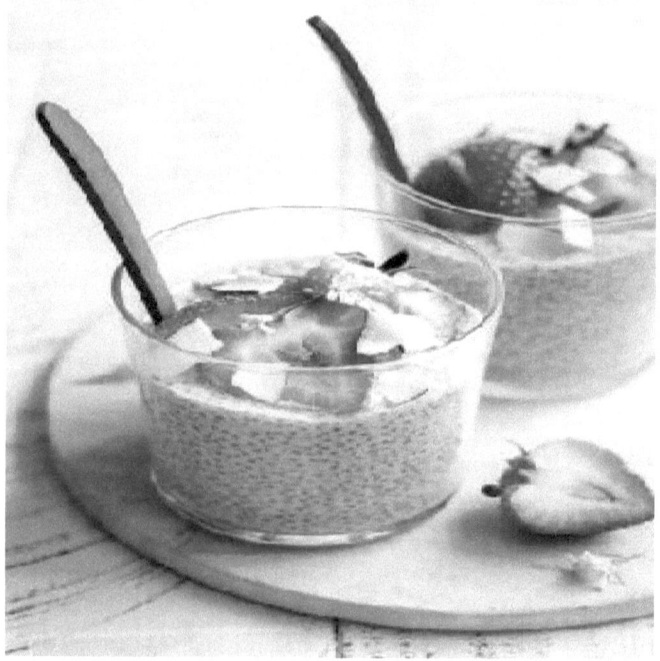

- SERVINGS: 1

<u>INGREDIENTS:</u>

- 200 ml almond milk
- 6 goji berries

- 4 tablespoons chia seeds

- 0.5 teaspoon cinnamon

- Sweetness like xylitol or erythritol

INSTRUCTIONS:

- Just put all the ingredients (except the goji berries) in a bowl and let it swell for about 2 hours, but also over night.

- Then spread the Goji berries and enjoy!

21. Low carb recipe for stuffed tuna eggs

Stuffed tuna eggs are popular party snacks. But even as a refined salad side dish they can do a lot. The nutritional value of tuna speaks for itself: 100g of tuna have a protein content of 24g. In addition, tuna contains 53g water and 0g carbohydrates - which makes tuna a popular food in the low carb diet .

- SERVINGS: 4 PEOPLE

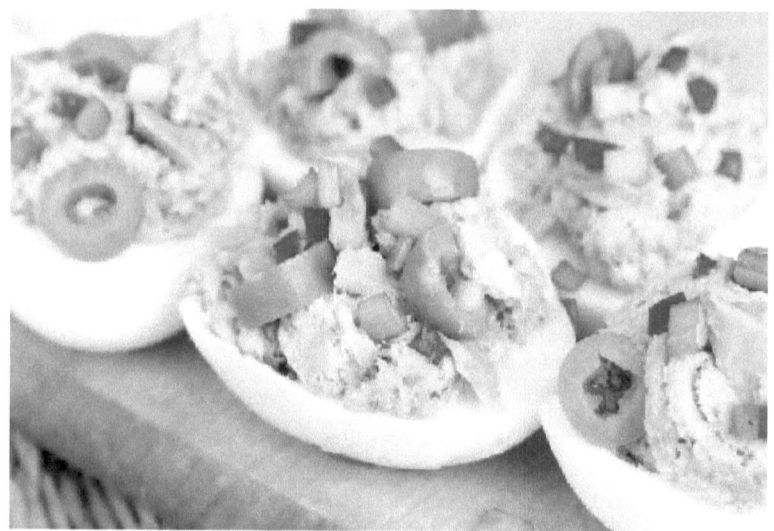

INGREDIENTS:

- 8 eggs cooked hard
- 140 g tuna
- 240 g mayonnaise
- Onion very finely chopped, 1 tbsp. For each egg
- Celery very finely chopped, 1 egg per egg
- salt
- pepper

INSTRUCTIONS:

- Halve the boiled eggs
- remove the egg yolk and mix with the remaining ingredients to a creamy mass.

- Then fill the egg halves with the mass.

- Finished!

Frequently asked questions

✓ How long does it take to get to Ketose?

A ketogenic diet is not a diet that can be stopped and restarted at any time. It takes some time for your body to get used to so-called ketosis. It takes between 2 and 7 days to reach this stage. It depends on your body, your level of activity and your diet. The quickest way to get into ketosis is to exercise on an empty stomach, limit your carb intake to 20 grams per day, and be alert to your water intake.

✓ Do I have to count calories?

At the end of the day, the calories count. Just make sure you eat properly. Prevent you from eating bad foods and do not let the deficit get too big.

During a keto diet you never have to worry about your calories. Because the fats and proteins will saturate you and bring a long-lasting satiety. But when you train, you have to be vigilant. With training, of course, comes a major calorie deficit and you have to eat to compensate for this again.

✓ Can I eat too much fat?

In short, yes, you can eat too much fat. The question before was about calories and why they are important. At the end of the day, we need a calorie deficit to lose weight. Too much fat will bring you over this deficit, which ends in extra calories. While it is very difficult for most people to overeat a low carb diet, it is theoretically possible.

✓ How much weight will I lose?

The weight loss you can achieve is entirely up to you. If you add sport to your diet, you will also lose more weight. Of course, if you banish fatteners from your diet, it helps. These include dairy products, sweeteners and wheat products.

Loss of weight due to lack of water is normal in a keto diet. Due to the dehydrating effect of the ketogenic diet you can lose a lot of weight within a few days. However, this is not fat that is lost. But it's a sign that your body is getting used to the ketogenic diet.

✓ How do I know that I am in ketosis?

The easiest way to tell if your body is in ketosis is by keto - sticks . These can be bought at the pharmacy. But you should keep in mind that these sticks are not 100% safe. They're more likely to give you an idea of whether you're in ketosis. Pink or purple on the stick indicate that ketones are being produced in your body. Dark colors usually mean that your body is dehydrated and the ketone level in your urine is heavily concentrated.

Ketosticks measure the amount of acetone in your urine. For a more accurate indication of ketone levels, you must use a blood ketone knife. This will show you an exact amount of ketone in your blood and will not be affected by hydration.

If you have a blood ketone knife, here is a brief explanation.

- Light ketosis: 0.5 mmol / L - 0.8 mmol / L

- Mean ketosis: 0.9 mmol / L - 1.4 mmol / L

- Strong ketosis: 1.5 mmol / L - 3.0 mmol / L

✓ How does ketosis work?

Ketosis is a state our body enters when we do not consume carbohydrates. It's a way for our body to use fat as its primary source of energy. It's not only healthy, it's also more effective for our brains.

How do we get the energy from the fats? The ketosis stage allows the liver to break fats into molecules, called ketones. These ketones bring the energy we need.

✓ How does this lead to weight loss?

Due to the calorie deficit, since we do not eat enough to produce energy, our body has to attack the fat stores to gain energy.

If you are more interested in the scientific side then you should keep yourself informed about ketosis and ketones .

✓ What about heart attacks with all the fat?

The main fats we consume are saturated and unsaturated fats. Until recently, there was a consensus that saturated fats are a cause of strokes. But in the meantime, studies have proven that saturated fats not only can not be held responsible for strokes, they actually benefit from cholesterol levels. You can eat these fats without hesitation.

The unsaturated fats are a bit more complicated. There are two things to consider here. Unsaturated fats like margarine are unhealthy and include trans fats. These should be avoided as they can lead to heart disease. However, there are also unsaturated fats, for example in fish, which are very healthy and have a positive effect on the cholesterol level. So it's your job to separate the good from the bad fats.

✓ I have just started and feel terrible. What can I do?

It is quite normal that headaches occur at the beginning of a keto diet. That's because ketosis acts dehydrating on your body, which also means you have to use the toilet a lot more often. Along with the fact that your body burns the last glycogen stores, it leads to a small disaster. You spin electrolytes like crazy and you have to replace them.

Drink a lot of water and eat salt. For example, salty meals, bacon, salted nuts. These are good foods to go into ketosis and keep you together.

✓ Constipation. What can I do?

Also in your intestine it will be a bit unpleasant at the beginning of the keto diet. Here is a list of things that will help you when your gut goes crazy.

- Magnesium Supplement

- Drink plenty of water

- Eat a spoonful of coconut oil

- Give up nuts

- Try to eat chia seeds

- Drink coffee and tea

✓ I lose no more weight. What can I do?

A stop in weight loss is completely normal. This can be traced back to different things. You can also try a few things to lose weight again. This includes not eating certain foods and changing your meal routine.

Here is a list of things that can be done in this case.

- Give up dairy products

- Take more fat to you

- Take less carbs

- Do not eat nuts anymore

- Give up gluten products

- No sweeteners anymore

✓ I train regularly! Should I be worried?

There are two types of athletes. They lift the races and lift the weights. If you belong to the first group (running, cycling, marathon) then you need not worry. Studies show that endurance sports are not influenced by low carb diets.

However, it does look different when you train with weights. Carbohydrates help your performance and also help to regenerate your muscles after exercise. There are two options here.

First Chance: A ketogenic diet in which you consume just enough carbohydrates to get out of the ketosis to get the workout done. After the training, you then go back into ketosis.

Second possibility: The cyclic ketogenic diet is a bit more complicated. This ketogenic diet is perfect for bodybuilding. You make the ketogenic diet for 5 days and then you increase your carbohydrate intake for 2 days.

✓ Which supplements should I consume?

Sometimes, when you start a keto diet, you may feel cramps or just not feel well. Here are some nutritional supplements that will help you get through the initial stages better.

- Multivitamin for women

- Multivitamin for men

- Magnesium Supplements

- Vitamin B supplement

- Vitamin D supplement

- Potassium supplement

Always contact your family doctor before you integrate vitamins and supplements into your diet.

Conclusion

A ketogenic diet can help to effectively reduce weight, but there are also critical opinions. Those considering a ketogenic diet should be well informed and undertake a diet change only in consultation with a physician and a nutritionist specializing in metabolic processes.

If you stick to the diet and completely dispense with carbohydrates, then you see after a short time first successes of the ketogenic diet. However, those who catch a free ticket for gulping up tons of meat and fat through the diet, the long-term plays with his health and will most likely not decrease, but even increase. As with all diets must be enjoyed here in moderation.

www.ingramcontent.com/pod-product-compliance
Lightning Source LLC
Chambersburg PA
CBHW051359280526
45784CB00007B/3022